THE GOALS AND THE DANGERS OF COVID VACCINES

(Bioethics)

THE GOALS AND THE DANGERS OF COVID VACCINES

(Bioethics)

Dr François Adja Assemien

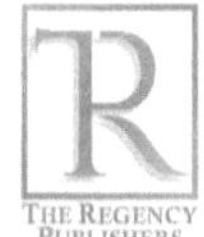

THE REGENCY PUBLISHERS

ISBN: 978-1-958517-95-6 (Paperback Edition)
ISBN: 978-1-958517-96-3 (Hardcover Edition)
ISBN: 978-1-958517-94-9 (E-book Edition)

Book Ordering Information

The Regency Publishers, US
521 5th Ave 17th floor NY, NY10175
Phone Number: (315)537-3088 ext 1007
Email: info@theregencypublishers.com
www.theregencypublishers.com

Printed in the United States of America

Contents

INTRODUCTION

The health crisis dubbed covid-19 leaves no one indifferent on earth. It affects everyone. It raises many questions. Indeed, it is the most tragic event of the century as a planetary catastrophe or genocide. This is the material that is causing the most saliva and ink to flow at the present time. It is the fashionable subject of thought, reflection and meditation for contemporary philosophers, sociologists and humanists. It is their fat cabbage. We must discuss this very seriously. We must constantly debate it in order to situate the duties and responsibilities of each other, in order to make people understand the stakes of this global scourge. Our time is going through its worst ordeal, the greatest crime against humanity or the most flagrant and cynical violation of all human rights. We must make people fully aware of all the dimensions and the dizzying depth of this general catastrophe. This moment is too serious and our priority must be given to this situation.

We must ask ourselves all the right questions that we must ask ourselves on this subject to get humans to reflect very seriously on their fate and on their history which is being done without them and **against them** .Nothing beats information. Nothing beats thought. Here we espouse Plato's theory of ascending and descending dialectics. We must do everything to enlighten and awaken all those who are still asleep and open the eyes to all the blind, to give sight to all myopic. We need to cure all schizophrenics. The good cause of humanity obliges it. The salvation of all men depends on it. We must mobilize and bring into combat all those who refuse to act, to see, to believe, to understand the infinite crimes happening on earth: covid-19, UN agenda 2021, new world order, eugenics , depopulation of earth, control of all humans, transhumanism, microchip in the body, vaccination passport, mass killing, terrorism, suppression of all rights and freedoms of peoples, destruction of jobs, businesses, savings everywhere. The overall stake of this book is to contribute to the happiness of humanity. And that necessarily goes through popular awareness, through general resistance and through everyone's struggle against the diabolical, satanic and demonic actions of globalists, eugenics, predators, oligarchs, Freemasons, imperialists. Our problem is as follows: who benefits from these multiple and infinite crimes against humanity? What should the victims do? Where is the world going? The rulers have ruined their countries. They have ruined the lives of their peoples. They have ruined everyone's joy of life. They turned peoples into prisoners. More seriously, they suppressed the fundamental rights of everyone with impunity .

In this book, we will outline the basic dangers and purposes of the corona virus and covid-19 vaccines. We identify two essential goals or dangers: planetary genocide and absolute control of humanity for financial gain. The planetary genocide has already started. It is very accelerated in Europe, Asia, America, Africa. The process of absolute, totalitarian control of all the inhabitants of the earth involves the compulsory vaccination of the seven billion of the world's population; hence the vaccine passport, the genetic identification of everyone thanks to electronics, 5 G, artificial intelligence. The goals are very closely related. They are combined, interdependent. They are mutually explained, dialectically. Each goal is in the other. Planetary genocide involves absolute control of humanity. All of this will be fully detailed in both parts of this book. The first part will deal with the slaughter of the masses. The second part will talk about the absolute control of humanity.

First Part

PLANETARY GENOCIDE

In the future it will be a question of finding a way to reduce the population. We will start with the old because as soon as he exceeds 60-65 years, man lives longer than he produces and he costs society dearly. Then the weak and then the useless ones who bring nothing to society because there will be more and more of them and mainly, finally, the stupid ones. Euthanasia targeting these groups; euthanasia will have to be an essential instrument of our future societies, in all cases. We will of course not be able to execute people or organize camps. We will get rid of it by making them believe that it is for their own good. Too large population, and for the most part unnecessary, is something economically too expensive. Socially, it is also much better for the human machine to come to an abrupt halt rather than gradually deteriorating . We won't be able to pass intelligence tests on millions and millions of people, you can imagine!

We will find something or cause it, a pandemic that targets certain people, a real economic crisis or not, a virus that will affect the old or the big, it doesn't matter, the weak will succumb to it, the fearful and the stupid will believe it and ask to be treated. We will have taken care to have planned the treatment, a treatment that will be the solution. The selection of idiots will thus be done by itself: they will go to the slaughterhouse of their own accord.

According to Jacques Attali, **L'Avenir de la vie** , 1981 (adviser to François Mittérand).

1

WHO ARE THE KILLERS?

The current planetary killers or genociders are all those who poison people around the world, who force covid-19 vaccines on the world's population. They are hired killers, white collar criminals. It is the Globalists, Eugenics, Freemasons, Illuminati, Transhumanists and Malthusians who rule the earth. They are present in all strata of society, in all activities and in all fields. They are everywhere. They manage and control all the states of the world politically, economically, financially, culturally, scientifically and militarily. They dictate their laws to them, impose their will on them. They carry out coups d'Etat against Presidents, Heads of State who resist them, who disobey them. They kill them and replace them with their lieges or submissive, docile, corrupt people (puppets, servants). These are the ultra-liberals, capitalists and oligarchs of all stripes. It is they who control international high finance, the big banks, international institutions like the World Bank, the International Monetary Fund , the World Health Organization, the United Nations, the European Union, the Club Bilderberg, ECOWAS, African Union, Club of Rome, NATO. Their names are: Adolphe Rothschild, John Davison Rockefeller, Jacques Attali, Nicolas Sarkozi, Emmanuel Macron, Bill and Melinda Gates ... There are also the owners of large pharmaceutical companies like GAVI, GSK, the real Masters of the world, who want create a new world order.

We can speak here of a dictatorship of the world's evil elite. This is, in particular, the case of the Great Reset. It is a world elite that wants to subdue all of humanity (Davos Forum). President Emmanuel Macron says: "The fates of an inhabitant of Rio, Legos, Canberra, Vienna, Paris, Dakar have never been so linked as they are today. Health, climate, inequalities, universal values: we need a global consensus, the same reading of the world, to unite our efforts to build together ". The former French President, Mr. Nicolas Sarkozi, said in a dictatorial and warlike tone: "No one will resist the new world order ... I mean no one". Everyone who fuels the fear of covid-19 and helps spread it (spread the lie) is a killer. **Fear kills** . It is responsible for this planetary tragedy. Anyone who believes in the reality of covid-19, the corona virus, is responsible for the tragedy. He is an accomplice of the executioners. He supports the planetary scam, lie and eugenics, imperialist and transhumanist conspiracy that is ravaging the world. He does so consciously (because of corruption) or for lack of information. All information agents, all politicians, all health workers, all doctors, all pharmacists, all zealous and devoted law enforcement officers (covidists) who fight and suppress protestors, rebels or **Whistleblowers** against **covidism** by calling them **conspirators** , liars are involved in the planetary genocide. They are executioners. All those who encourage and trick people into believing in covid-19 and getting vaccinated are criminals, unrepentant hitmen. They are in the camp of the enemies, of the Freemasons, of the Covidists, of the globalists, of the eugenics, of the transhumanists as supporters of the new world order. They are enemies of humanity. They do so either out of ignorance or skepticism or out of constraint or out of self-interest (corruption).

They are at the service of the devil, of lucifer. All are guilty of the planetary genocide. This is, in particular, the case of journalists, communication officers, political leaders (Presidents, Heads of State, Ministers, Representatives, Mayors, Ambassadors, Senators), civil servants, employers , employees, workers, police officers. Covid-19 propaganda and the belief in the corona virus are self-interested and remunerated by the world's evil political and economic elite (ultra-liberal and capitalist oligarchy). This criminal elite relies on all those who are corruptible, weak in character, light-hearted, oblivious, ignorant and irresponsible to spread the lie about the existence of covid-19, to keep the fear panic in the world. This catastrophic fear serves them to suppress all the freedoms and all the fundamental rights of men in order to impose their new world order. So in the name of the fear of covid-19, men obediently and willingly accept liberticidal measures and alienate all their rights to a minority of oppressors, predators, dictators wanting to subdue and control the whole world. Finally, the killers and their associates around the world are all those who protect, defend and keep alive the deceitful and criminal covid-19 system. They are the masters, the powerful, the executioners, the slaves, the weak, the sheep or all those who are resigned. The only worthy, responsible, innocent beings are the resistance fighters whom we call rebels. They alone are free and independent in the world. We therefore distinguish three categories of people on earth: the **executioners** (masters, lions, oligarchs, capitalists, eugenists, transhumanists, globalists), **victims** (dominated, slaves, sheep, weak, docile, resigned) and **rebels** (launchers of alert, awakening consciousness, sheep friends).

The phenomenon of covid-19 is a fierce planetary war, the third world war, silent with soft weapons (poisons, sprays, virus, 5 G, fear, vaccines). Let's call it **covidism**. Covidism is a capitalist, oligarchic, Freemasonic, globalist, political, economic, social, cultural, philosophical, scientific, technological, mystical crime (the Great Reset). It is a global and totalitarian system. It is the secret, insidious war waged by the strong, the powerful and the plutocrats around the world against the people and the weak. All the Malthusian Presidents of the world are killers of their peoples. They apply the lesson of Malthus: **limit births, decrease the world population, increase food production to avoid famines due to overpopulation** . The neo-Malthusians make the limitation of births a human right and a human duty

---

(the biotic law passed in France under President Emmanuel Macron). Hence the mandatory, fatal, sterilizing and anti-natalist vaccinations. Neo-Malthusianism and Covidism are the main sources of eugenics and transhumanism. Let us summarize the political, economic and social thought of Thomas Robert Malthus: the demographic progression is faster than the increase in resources, hence the impoverishment of the population. Wars and epidemics (famine, black plague, flu ...) regulate demography. The covid-19 ravaging the earth today is therefore timely. There must be more food than mouths to feed. Economic growth (increase in resources) must be greater than population growth. This is the condition for the happiness and salvation of mankind. This implies and leads to birth control, the drastic reduction of the world population by covidism (see Jacques Attali).

All the means to achieve this end are good. The end justifies the means here. And means implies right. It is Machiavellianism and cynicism. Malthus predicted that the population size will decrease to zero if the death rate is greater than the birth rate, and will increase to infinity if the birth rate is greater than the death rate. Malthus aims to regulate and control the growth of the population. In his work entitled "Essay on the principle of populations", he shows that there is an asymmetry between the growth of the population and the growth of the production of resources. And according to him, if no effort is made to balance these two things, demographic catastrophe will be inevitable. This is a doctrinal or theoretical origin of covid-19. Covidism is explained at the same time by Malthusianism, Machiavellianism and Attalism.

2

THE REASONS OF THE PLANETARY GENOCIDE

Why are people committing planetary genocide? What is genocide? Genocide is an act of wickedness and extreme barbarism. It consists in massacring, exterminating a people, an ethnic group, a group etc. This particular case, the most serious in human history as the extermination of humanity, can be explained by three fundamental objective reasons. The first is socio-economic. We attribute it to Thomas Robert Malthus (English economist) and Nicolas Machiavelli (Italian philosopher). It is Malthusianism and Machiavellianism. Malthus has shown that when a couple's bed is too fruitful, their table is thin. It is the same with a country and the whole world. Indeed, demographic growth (very large population) represents a danger for countries because it leads to economic ruin, poverty and famine. Indeed, it is very difficult for each country to be able to feed, maintain, manage and satisfy an overabundant population when its economic resources are weak or insufficient. Each state must make its subjects happy by providing for their basic needs. It must provide them with decent housing, work, food, schools, hospitals, roads, security etc. Malthus' lesson to the rulers of the world says to balance the growth of population with the growth of economic output. Better still, **economic growth must be greater than demographic**

growth . This leads incompetent rulers who like ease, who cannot make their subjects happy, to want to kill them, to reduce their populations. This is called the depopulation or depopulation of a country. It is a shortcut thanks to eugenics, to transhumanism (the French biotic and anti-natalist law). Incapable, lazy and irresponsible rulers (Emmanuel Macron and others) prefer to decrease their populations through covidism and other criminal means. It is a global scourge today. This is the socio-economic source of planetary genocide and universal covidism.

We notice that where people die the most from covid-19 and mass **compulsory vaccinations** are the countries that are quite or very populated, with very cynical, Machiavellian, Malthusianist, Freemason, globalist leaders. These are countries which have an interest in reducing their populations and which do everything to ensure that as many people as possible die or rather are killed (terrifying logic of the vaccine dynamic). The leaders of these countries want to do everything to achieve their macabre goals with their formidable and absolutely effective weapon that is covidism (brilliant find or invention of the century). Think of the famous vaccine passport which is in force in France against thick and thin. Think about the phenomenon of yellow vests in France. Think of President Emmanuel Macron's historic and very cynical speech: "The beast is here. It comes...". Think of the biotic law passed in France etc. **So covidism will never end on earth** . The world will go from bad to worse, from variant to variant ad aeternam. The covidist rulers, plotters and globalists do not bother with morals or humanism to commit genocide against their peoples. They will stop at nothing to slaughter with impunity and gleefully their innocent, naive fellow citizens. They are very determined and resolute. They use all means (violent and gentle): spraying, pollution of the air and the atmosphere, 5 G, climate modification, poisons of all kinds, drugs, vaccines ... The end justifies the means.

The second objective reason for the planetary genocide is political. The globalist elite, made up of Freemasons, bosses, owners of pharmaceutical companies, scientists, doctors, politicians, bankers, businessmen and others, want to form a collectivist and authoritarian world government (bloodthirsty dictatorship of ultra-liberals, capitalists and mystics). This planetary government will replace all the governments of the world. It will wrest the independence and sovereignty of all the states of earth. It will vassalize all the political leaders of the world. It is it alone that will manage all the goods and all the riches of earth (the world economy) and will administer all mankind. It will change humanity, civilization, nature and the universe through science and technology. It will use artificial intelligence to recreate humanity, animals, life, flora, modify the climate (cooling the earth). So the humans of the future will be very strange beings, zombies made from scratch in laboratories (mixed with animals) who will act like robots. Man will therefore be denatured, dehumanized, alienated, mechanized. It will be a simple instrument that can be manipulated at will and absolutely submissive. They will put an electronic chip in his body which will have its perverting and harmful effect by making him controllable anywhere and at any time. This human will be devoid of reason, intelligence, feeling, emotion, lucidity, desire, morality, humanism, personality, will, in short, humanity. He will not act but will be acted upon. Marriage between man and woman will be prohibited. There will be no more family (father, mother, child), no more parental, familial, natural attachment (Platonism in **La République**). There will no longer be the right to procreate naturally but only by scientific methods. People will be sterilized.   The world government will manufacture and impose a digital single currency on all of the earth. The identity of each person will be digitized and connected to a computer network thanks to the electronic chip placed in the body of each individual. The world government will take care of feeding, housing, dressing, maintaining, caring for everyone for free (communism). Because it exclusively holds all the rights, all the goods and all the individual, collective and state powers of the world in economic, political, social, cultural, spiritual, intellectual, scientific, technological matters. Machines, robots, drones will do all the work instead of humans (artificial intelligence).

The third reason (or motive) of the planetary genocide is of a purely spiritual, religious, mystical order. They want to establish an absolute authority of the Freemasons, the Illuminati and others on the whole world. It is about consecrating, consolidating and confirming the total and absolute power of these spiritual and religious masters in the world. Hence this war for the creation of a world government and a new world order or a new world normal. It is totalitarianism and mystico-religious imperialism of the Freemasons against Judeo-Christianity and other spiritual and religious movements of the earth. Freemasonry is defined by Le Petit Robert as "... An esoteric and initiatory association, of a philosophical and progressive nature, which is dedicated to the search for truth, to the improvement of man and society" . It is therefore a movement which claims to be humanist but which is above all transhumanist, elitist and eugenic. For Freemasons, means implies right. Current science and technology make it possible to artificially recreate man in laboratories. Artificial intelligence is called upon to transform humanity. Thus President Emmanuel Macron, a great Freemason, recently passed a law in France entitled **the biotic law which removes the border between the human species and the animal species**. This law allows human fetuses to be mixed with animal fetuses to give birth to a new species to be made from both human and animal. What a monstrosity! This same biotic law authorizes "infanticide". From now on we can kill a child who is in his mother's womb. Women can terminate their nine-month pregnancies . In other words, the French government encourages abortion or the killing of babies. In short, France does not want any more children. It is the reduction of the population at the base. This is in the agenda of the new world order of eugenic and transhumanist globalists. This agenda requires the suppression of natural procreation through sexual intercourse between man and woman. It forbids attachment and family. Paternity and the physical father of a child are now considered unnecessary. It is about separating the children from their fathers. Plato's utopia (in **The Republic**) is becoming reality in the world today.

Science and technology are responsible for artificially making abnormal beings, hybrids, obedient zombies like machines, robots to use, to dominate, to command. Economically, this is very profitable for the capitalists. Politically, this is very interesting for the ruling oligarchs, absolutists and globalists. This clearly shows their desire for domination and all-out power. Science and technology thus affirm and confirm their prodigious and immoral progress. This is exacerbated, outrageous scientism. Bioethics has work to do here. These are the causes or the origins of covid-19 as a weapon or means of depopulation of earth for the benefit of the capitalist oligarchy and the eugenicist and Freemasonry globalist elite (Jacques Attali, Rockefeller, Rothschild, Malthus, Bill Gates, Georges Soros, Emmanuel Macron ...). It is the Great Reset that benefits all corrupt governments on earth. Sterilization, abortion, poisoning, covid-19 and compulsory mass vaccinations constitute the instruments of the depopulation of earth desired by the globalists. People all over the world, wake up. Stand up. Let us fight together so that the will of the globalist executioners cannot be achieved to our detriment. Let us all fight to death the realization of their new satanic world order, their new demonic normal. Let's refuse their vaccines.

3

THE PLANETARY GENOCIDE MODE

How does the planetary genocide operate? The political, economic and financial elite which govern the world are massacring the weak, the powerless and the peoples in a sly, hypocritical, secret war. This war works by cunning, Machiavellianism, Malthusianism, cynicism, eugenics, transhumanism. It is based on selfishness, self-centeredness, biotechnology and nanotechnology. The neo-liberal, ultra-capitalist and globalist oligarchy uses all means to achieve its end which is the "new normal". This is summed up by the concept of the Grand Reset or New World Order. It includes the demise of democracies, health dictatorship (health passport), techno-surveillance, confinement. The Great Reset is both a political, economic and social prospecting book published in July 2020, an Agenda and a conspiracy theory. This book is signed by two eminent members of the World Economic Forum in Davos. Their names are: klaus Schwab (economist) who is the founder and Thierry Malleret (economist) who was the director. For the authors of The Great Reset, the covid-19 pandemic "represents a rare but narrow window of opportunity to reflect, reimagine and reset our world."

The New World Order is a formula used to refer to several conspiracy theories. These theories denounce a plan for planetary domination through supposedly democratic institutions, non-governmental institutions or even totalitarian regimes. Some proponents of this conspiracy theory appeal to hypothetical groups such as the Illuminati and denounce a vast, centuries-old conspiracy. World events would thus be orchestrated by a group of individuals acting in the shadows, bearers of a long-standing totalitarian project. The groups designated as the conspirators vary widely between versions. Real groups, secret societies or the business world, are referred to as the "brains" behind this vast secret project of world control: elitist international organizations and foundations such as the Council on Foreign Relations, the Trilateral Commission, the group Bilderberg, the Club of Rome, the Ditchley Foundation or closed groups like Freemasons, Skull and Bones, Bohemian Club, Ordo Templi Orientis etc.

Covid-19 is a code or acronym. It means: Certificate of vaccination Identity. 19: 1 means A; 9 stands for I. The whole stands for Artificial Intelligence. Clearly, covid-19 stands for Vaccine Identity Certificate based on artificial intelligence. It is therefore not the name of a pandemic (disease). It is a secret code which sums up the whole criminal system of the Great Reset, of genocidal, eugenic transhumanism including fatal spreading, confinement, fear as a psychological weapon of submission of everyone and compulsory vaccinations of the masses causing death and general sterilization. What is covid-19? Google tells us that it is a new disease caused by a new corona virus that has never been seen in humans. A new corona virus is a corona virus that has never been identified. The virus causing corona virus 2019 disease (covid-19) is not the same as the corona viruses that are commonly transmitted to humans and cause minor illnesses such as a common cold. Covid-19: how is it transmitted? The virus is considered to be transmitted mainly from person to person:

-Between people close to each other (less than two meters)

-Via respiratory droplets that are expelled when an infected person coughs, sneezes or speaks. These droplets can get into the mouth or nose of people around and even be inhaled into the lungs. People without symptoms can transmit covid-19. Symptoms of covid-19 can include:

-fever

-cough
-breathing difficulties
-chills
-muscle aches
-sore throat
-new loss of taste or smell
 It may take 2 to 14 days for symptoms to appear.

Potential complications of covid-19

* Covid-19 disease can take a moderate or severe form.
* Severe cases of covid-19 can lead to complications, including pneumonia.
* Covid-19 can cause death in people with severe illness and lead to complications.

People at high risk of serious illness from covid-19

People of all ages with underlying health problems, especially if these problems are poorly controlled, including people with:
    * Chronic lung disease or moderate to severe asthma
    * Serious heart problems
    * A weakened immune system
    * Severe obesity (body mass index (BMI) of 40 or more)
    * Diabetes
    * Chronic kidney disease, especially with dialysis
    * Liver disease

How To Prevent Covid-19: Message To Get Across

Practice social distancing and be sure to wash your hands. Sacred texts can help communicate prevention messages among religious communities.
    * Wash your hands often with soapy water for at least 20 seconds.

- If soap and water are not available, you can use an alcohol-based hand sanitizer with at least 60% alcohol.

- If you do not have access to soap or disinfectant, use a chlorine-based solution (water and bleach)

* Do not touch your eyes, nose and mouth with unwashed hands.

What is spreading?

It is the pollution of the air and the atmosphere that promotes the spread of viral diseases. Agricultural spraying is accused of worsening symptoms of covid-19. A recent study from the University of Havard showed that fine particle pollution increased covid-19 mortality by 15%.

Second Part

THE ABSOLUTE CONTROL OF HUMANITY

We will put in place a monetary system that will make them prisoners forever and that will put their children in fault and in debt. We will focus their attention on money and material possessions so that many never connect with their inner selves. We will use soft metals, aging accelerators and tranquilizers in food and water and also in the air. The metals will cause them to lose their intelligence. It is therefore alluminium, copper etc. We promise to find an antidote in our many fields . And we'll feed them with more poisons. The toxins will be absorbed through their skins and mouths destroying their brain and reproductive system. The toxins will be hidden in everything around them, in what they drink, eat, breathe and wear. With funny pictures and music, they will be taught that poisons are good. When women give birth, we will inject toxins into the blood of their children and convince them that it is to help them. We'll start as soon as possible when their brains are still young. We will take their children with what they love, sugar. When their ability to learn is reduced, we will create drugs that will make them even sicker and cause other diseases for which we will create more drugs. We will use our power to make them docile and weak. They will grow up being depressed, sluggish, and overweight. We will distract them with sexual immorality, pleasures and games. They will do what we tell them. If they resist us, we will find ways to use consciousness- changing technologies in their lives . We will use fear as our weapon. We will build their governments by creating animosities within them. We will have both sides. They will do the work for us and we will thrive on their debts and hard work. If we like, we'll have them kill each other. We will control all aspects of their life and tell them what and how to think. They will be busy killing each other until our ultimate goal is reached. We will continue to make them live in fear and anger over picture and sound and so on.

1

WHO CONTROLS HUMANITY?

Humanity is controlled by masters, leaders and gurus. It is found in the shepherd-to-flock relationship. The masters are the philosophers, scientists, technicians, businessmen, mystics, politicians and others. When it comes to corona virus, covid-19, and covid vaccines, the masters who control the world are well known. At their head are thinkers, philosophers, elites oligarchs, economists, businessmen, mystics, Freemasons, transhumanists and progressives. The controllers of humanity are all those who act for the change or transformation of humanity. They claim to improve the nature, condition and life of men in the world. They refuse man as he is with his natural and historical attributes. They want his artificial recreation. For them, means implies right. Their means are science and technology. They are eugenics. Medicine, biology, information technology, nanotechnology, artificial intelligence, genetics and genetic engineering are doing great things. They succeed in making man, in controlling his thinking, his feelings, his emotions, his health, his movements. These philosophers want to create a new world order, a new normal. They manifest themselves in the political, economic, mystical fields. This is the case of President Emmanuel Macron, a transhumanist, who passed **a biotic law** . This is also the case with people like Malthus (economist), Jacques Attali (adviser to President François

Mitterand), billionaire Georges Soros, Bill Gates, John Davidson Rockefeller, Adolph Rothschild.

They are grouped together in various associations for economic, political, scientific, technological, mystical and medical purposes. There are the members of The Grand Reset, the Bilderberg Club, Big Pharma, WHO, OMC, GAVI, GSK, UN, World Bank, International Monetary Fund, European Union, Club of Rome, African Union, ECOWAS, UNICEF, NATO. It is an ultra-capitalist oligarchy. In order to supposedly improve the condition and health of mankind, it manufactures medicines. It has just hastily developed dubious, disputed, hypothetical vaccines called Oxford Astra Zeneca (or Vaxzevria), Pfizer-Biontech (or Comirnaty), Moderna (or Spikevax), Janssen (or Johnson). In the opinion of the creators of these vaccines (which in fact do not meet the necessary and sufficient conditions for authentic vaccines), humanity will be saved thanks to their findings, to their products. But it is clear that it is these fake vaccines that are killing, poisoning, crippling, paralyzing many people on earth. It is even said that anyone who is vaccinated will die for sure after two years. Because the side effects of these pseudo-vaccines on their guinea pigs are terrible and unbearable. The bodies of vaccinated people have become a magnet that holds cell phones to their arms. That is to say that these vaccines absolutely contain terrible things which make it possible to control the vaccinated "guinea pigs" (nanoparticles !?). Isn't the unacknowledged, secret goal of these fake vaccines to allow the drastic reduction of the world population, that is to say the depopulation of earth so dear to the supporters of the new world order?

What do globalists, who are transhumanists and eugenics, want to control? They seek to control humanity, i.e. thought, feelings, emotions, movements, health, education, politics, culture, communication, media, spirituality, religion, economy, money, goods, riches of the earth. They want to make it all their own. They want to own the world, to transform man and things to their liking, their needs and their fancies. They want to dominate humanity, nature, universe. To achieve their ends, they create poisons, drugs, fake vaccines, deadly gene therapy, sterilizers, zombies, robotic men, drones, artificial intelligence. It is called eulogistically and emphatically, without any shame or moral scruples "the new normal" (the new world order). It is the secret war against all the ignorant, weak, helpless, defenseless peoples of the earth. "The rulers have ruined our countries, have ruined our lives, have ruined our joy of living, have transformed us into prisoners and above all have suppressed our fundamental rights with impunity, without being disturbed in any way."

The masters who control humanity and the world employ effective scientific and technological means such as cloning, assisted reproduction, curettage, genetic testing, gene therapy, euthanasia, eugenics, cell research strains, organ donation, surrogacy.

2

THE REASONS FOR ABSOLUTE CONTROL OF HUMANITY

The reasons for the absolute control of humanity by the oligarchy or the world elite are manifold. The main reason is the desire for domination and all-out power. To govern or to lead is also to control. But here, it is a question of suppressing all the freedoms and all the fundamental rights of humanity as a whole. The globalists want to reduce each human being to his simplest expression by transforming him into a baby. They try to denature him, to alienate him, to strip him completely and to follow him step by step everywhere and at all times. We try to deprive him of all his powers, all his capacities to think, to want, to decide, to criticize, to judge, to reflect, to challenge, to protest, to refuse, to say no. It is about the establishment of a global policy that will transform every human being into a robot as a remote-controlled thing or instrument. To control men in this way is to prevent them from living, thinking and acting naturally according to their will as free, autonomous, responsible, sovereign beings. It is about making them transparent, to be able to read their thoughts, their feelings, their emotions, to modify their mind and to get them to think, to feel, to act as one wants them to think, feel and act (beings manipulable, robotic). It is, in fact, to dispose of the life of each individual on earth, to make him a slave or a child without the right to speak out or to historical, political, economic, social, ethical initiatives. The globalists want to make him accept unacceptable things, decisions, laws, a new normal or a new world order that is completely arbitrary, unjust, illegitimate, criminal, inhuman. The unrepentant globalist dictators and executioners impose their paradigm, their vision of humanity, of the world and of life on others. It is their geopolitics and their geo-economy.

The second reason for controlling humanity is geo-economic. The controllers of humanity are businessmen. They are sellers of drugs, vaccines, industrialists, technicians, statesmen who want to exploit the goods and the riches of earth. They are looters, oligarchs, neoliberals and capitalists. People like Bill Gates, Georges Soros, Davidson Rockefeller, Jacques Attali, Adolphe De Rothschild have an interest in controlling health, thinking, feelings, emotions, movement, education, governments, economies, cultures, the goods and riches of earth (IMF, WHO, WTO, GAVI, GSK, UN, WB, UNICEF, European Union, Paris Club, Club of Rome, Club Bilderberg, Big Pharma, The Great Reset). Indeed, it is their reason for living and their reason for being. They trample, violate blithely and with impunity the laws of bioethics. They benefit from the current catastrophic system or the new world order. It is their doing. Transhumanism, vaccines, covid-19 are their facts. Geopolitics and geo-economics are accompanied by geo-militarization and geo-strategy which are the basis of slavery, colonization, imperialism, wars. "The real power is military," said Alain (French philosopher). Slavery, colonization and imperialism are possible thanks to military power. The liberation, decolonization, independence and sovereignty of an occupied, invaded country are also possible through military power. The case of the formerly occupied, colonized countries, which liberated themselves, decolonized thanks to their bravery and their military power is very edifying here. USA, France, Algeria, Vietnam, Angola, Cuba, Zimbabwe, Ethiopia etc. are among these countries.

The plan for the new world order is already known. The advantages of the globalists are exorbitant, very colossal. Compulsory vaccination of the earth's seven billion inhabitants is underway all over the world. Their side effects are death, gene or genetic transformation of all humans, systematic sterilization of people. There are already thousands or millions of deaths that are hidden from us. The goal of this compulsory vaccination of the masses being the physical suppression of 80% of the world population (at the very least), there will soon be only a tiny minority of people on earth. The latter will be transhumanized (see transhumanism and the biotic law passed in France under President Emmanuel Macron). If the depopulation of earth succeeds, to whom will all the goods and all the riches of the world go? It will logically and rightfully come to those who kill others, to predators or globalist executioners. It will be up to the rulers and controllers of earth alone. This will fall to the tyrannical world government that will soon be formed (presumably the UN with the World Bank and NATO). All the countries of the world are asked to give up their sovereignty and cede it willingly or by force to the collectivist world government which is on the horizon. Malthus' genocidal economic theory is already in application and in force around the world. It consists of drastically reducing the population of each country and increasing the growth of economic production to supposedly avoid famine, poverty, misery in the world. This is how the globalists want to create the conditions for the happiness of humanity which will be dehumanized, animalized and objectified. This represents the worst cynicism and the worst Machiavellianism ever achieved in the history of mankind. This is not a problem for the transhumanists, mystics, wizards and demons dressed as human beings who rule all the countries of the world. A President or Head of State who dares to oppose this new world order is immediately killed or overthrown by a coup. These assassinations are legion in Africa in recent years. To this globalist end, rulers, health personnel, journalists and other authorities or officials in other fields are paid a high price. They are paid dearly to bring death and misfortune to mankind. We are therefore in the dynamics and logic of the mafia and mercenarism. Some have the role of killing and others have the role of lying to people, forcing them to believe in covid-19 and fostering fear of covid-19. This is the system we call **covidism.** Let us quote Mr. Jacques Attali, great theorist of this criminal situation: "In the future it will be a question of finding a way to reduce the population. We will start with the old, because as soon as he exceeds 60-65 years, man lives longer than he produces and he costs society dearly. Then the weak and then the useless ones who bring nothing to society because there will be more and more of them and finally the stupid ones. Euthanasia targeting these groups; euthanasia will have to be an essential instrument of our future societies in all cases. We will of course not be able to execute people or organize camps. We will get rid of it by making them believe it is for their own good. A too large population, and for the most part unnecessary, is something economically too expensive. Socially, it is also much better for the human machine to come to an abrupt halt rather than gradually deteriorating. We won't be able to pass intelligence tests on millions and millions of people, you can imagine!

We will find something or cause it, a pandemic that targets certain people, a real economic crisis or not, a virus that will affect the old or the big, it doesn't matter, the weak will succumb to it, the fearful and the stupid will believe and ask to be treated. We will have taken care to have planned the treatment, a treatment that will be the solution. The selection of idiots will thus be done by itself: they will go of their own accord to the slaughterhouse "(in **L'Avenir de la vie** , 1981). Mr. Jacques Attali wrote this book when he was adviser to President François Mitterand in France. Is not this Malthusian, elitist, eugenic and genocidal Agenda implemented on earth? What do the masquerade, the lie, the mishmash, the intrigues, the plot and the Machiavellianism of covidism represent? Mr. Jacques Attali speaks of provoked pandemic, viruses, drugs, transhumanism, violation of bioethics, lies, deception, conspiracy. He proposed heinous crimes against humanity. Which presidential adviser?

3

THE MODE OF HUMANITY CONTROL

It is the control of all humans and all properties. What are the instruments? The economic system by which the globalists control the world (they manage and exploit all the wealth of earth) is called capitalism or economic liberalism. This made it possible to set up private commercial companies in all the capitalist countries. These are sometimes grouped together and form what are called multinational corporations that exploit the goods, wealth, natural and mineral resources of Third World countries. They dominate governments and control their economies. They intervene in the socio-political and socio-economic life of the countries in which they have settled comfortably and durably. Multinationals wage wars and coups d'Etat against Heads of State, Patriotic Presidents, just, honest, who are hostile to them, who oppose their abuses and exactions: predation, corruption, injustice, arbitrariness, oppression, exploitation of man by man, terrorism, deterioration of the terms of trade. Supported by their imperialist countries, these multinationals impose dishonest, corrupt, traitors, puppets, servants and accomplices of Western imperialism on the weak and underdeveloped countries of the Third World. Thus these multinational companies exercise a ferocious dictatorship and a Machiavellianism of the most cynical in the world. This is how they make very big profits like leeches, vampires and deadly parasites. They ruin, impoverish the Third World. They implicitly govern all the countries of the Third World.

The World Bank, IMF and other similar institutions lend money at exorbitant interest rates to weak, poor, powerless countries. These donors are over-indebting and strangling small countries. If the latter fail to repay their debts to them, they confiscate and exploit their properties, their strategic natural and mining resources such as gold, diamonds, uranium, petroleum, cobalt, iron, agricultural products (coffee, cocoa, pineapple, bananas, rubber, etc.). It becomes their private properties as hostages. So there are neo-slavery, neo-colonized, proletarianized and alienated countries nowadays in Africa, America, Europe and Asia etc. The capitalist, predatory and imperialist oligarchy has its grip on them. These are its hunting grounds, its colonial enclosures or its trading posts.

This same imperialist oligarchy also uses religion and mysticism to control humanity. It thus atrophies the spirit of humanity. It is spiritual slavery or colonization. This is the role of missionaries, priests, pastors, Imams, gurus in the world. Religion and mysticism constitute a real psychological opium, a moral and mental danger against peoples (Karl Marx). Indeed, they make renuncers by turning the gaze of naive, gullible, drugged peoples towards the clouds and the sky and by promoting hypocritical predation, the systematic plundering of the real and concrete goods and riches of earth (see the message of the King Leopold II of Belgium to his missionaries in the Congo and the ill-gotten fortune of the Vatican). Science and technology also allow the globalist capitalist oligarchy to control humanity very effectively. These are biology, the information industry, nano-technology, medicine, virology, the arms industry, pharmacology. Corona virus, covid-19 pandemic, Ebola fever, AIDS and malaria, in short, most diseases are created by the laboratories that manufacture and sell drugs, vaccines. Bacteriology makes bacteria that serve as a weapon of mass destruction. Atomic and nuclear weapons allow their makers to subdue, to control the small, weak and powerless Third World countries. They promote the continued slavery and colonization of non-industrialized peoples and countries. The French philosopher, René Descartes, said that science and technology would make man as master and possessor of nature. This is verified today. It is the sad reality of the world. Science and technology have made the capitalist and globalist oligarchs the masters and owners not only of nature, earth, universe but also of humanity. It made executioners who exploit and slaughter humanity. Pharmacologists do not seek our good health, nor our happiness. They seek their profits at the expense of our health. We are their guinea pigs and their laboratory mice (false covid-19 vaccines). They sell their drugs and vaccines to get as rich as possible by poisoning and killing billions of people on earth. The inventors of health products and vaccines are undertakers. They are creators of diseases and pandemics that are very lucrative for them (business). The French with their Instituts Pasteur in the world are very prosperous. GAVI, GSK, Big Pharma, OMS, Bill Gates, Rockefeller, Georges Soros are also. The supporters of transhumanism, the new world order and the 5 G are in the same condition. This is how the real false anti-covid-19 vaccines and other health products are multiplying ad infinitum and are imposed manu militari on everyone. It is a very lucrative and very prosperous business for the capitalist oligarchs, cynics, Machiavellians, Malthusianists, Platonists, "Attalists" (Jacques Attali). All means are good for these executioners. Provoking endless health crises and catastrophic pandemics (such as global genocide) is child's play for them. It is also their safest and most effective way to obtain unexpected economic growth as an end in itself and for itself (Jacques Attali and Malthus).

CONCLUSION

We are talking about humanity. For us, this is the greatest value and the end in itself. So we invite everyone to the fight that will defend, protect and save humanity. We must save the life of humanity which is currently in danger. It is about the terrible danger of its **disappearance**. Those who work for the disappearance of humanity are known. They are well identified. It is the global neo-liberal elite or the capitalist oligarchs. These are the globalist transhumanists. We know their egoistic, egocentric, eugenic and hegemonic motives. We know their very formidable and powerful weapons. It is science and technology that allow them to manufacture diseases, pandemics, viruses, bacteria (Ebola, AIDS, corona virus, Covid-19 ...) as silent weapons to wage an atrocious, secret, endless war to the peoples. These enemies of humanity are destroying the civilization that gave us birth and growth in good health, which gave us normal, happy, healthy lives. These **mad** and barbaric enemies are replacing civilization with barbarism, with their diabolical, satanic utopia of wizards, demons, mystics and anti-natalist philosophers, eugenics, elitists, transhumanists. This criminal utopia as a distorting, destructive, tragic, murderous vision of humanity, of life is paradoxically and ironically called the *new normal* (supreme and murderous madness). We must therefore redefine ethics, eudemonism and axiology. We must redefine the philosophy and the moral notions of progress, civilization, good, evil, happiness, person, normality, value, humanism, humanity. This moment is really serious. Everything is called into question. It is the most terrible revolution as an intellectual and moral cataclysm in history. Order has become disorder and disorder has become order. Abnormality has become normality and normality has become abnormality. Good has become evil and evil has become good. Wisdom has become madness and madness has become wisdom. Happiness has become unhappiness and unhappiness has become happiness. We will have seen it all. You lose all your Latin. Where are we going to ? Are we heading towards which world? Is it time for the transvaluation of all the values of which Nietzsche spoke? Is this the genealogy of morals? Are we already beyond Good and Evil?

This crazy dream that is being carried out all over the world is not without motives and causes. It reflects the will of globalists, predators, executioners to control humanity and to dispose of the earth and the universe. Humanity is facing a veritable silent third world war. Financial, spiritual, religious, scientific, technical, intellectual and political powers wage war on humanity and civilization. What to do? The peoples of earth must wake up from their too long sleep which only favors their domination, their oppression and their massacre. They have to stand up and go on the defensive at least. **They must use their right to self-defense.** They do that or it is everyone's death. All those who will have the chance to read this book will have the duty to inform others, to open their eyes. We must make sure that all deaf hear our message, that all blind people now see clearly, that all ignorant people become knowledgeable. All the dominated and all the victims must become rebels, revolutionaries. All sheep must become indomitable lions. All earthworms must become ferocious beasts. Let us all be skeptical from now on, people who do not believe in anything coming from the globalist rulers, covidists, the dishonest media, the corrupt media, in the pay of the executioners. Protect our right to freedom, to health, to life, to our sovereignty, to well-being, to security, to peace, to happiness, to truth, to justice. These values are sacred. They are not negotiable. They are inalienable. Let us love each other, unite, stand in solidarity, march and protest together, democratically, legally and legitimately. Prison is better than death. Prison without crime is glory. It is a means of our salvation. Let us condemn very strongly the genocidal tyranny and the arbitrary and unjust rule of man by man that is taking place all over the world. Let us all seek only the government of man through the law which is the expression of the general will.

We vigorously challenge and fight all unjust, harmful and arbitrary measures and decisions which condemn us to certain death. So-called anti-covid vaccines are products at the experimental stage. Their side effects are disastrous, catastrophic. These are deadly products in the short or medium term. They don't protect anyone against covid-19. Anyone who is vaccinated can be infected. He herself can infect others because he is vaccinated. He has poison in her body. He has become very dangerous. He is said to reproduce variants. His natural immune system is destroyed. What is the use of getting vaccinated? What are the advantages of these vaccines for the vaccinated? What then are the real and unacknowledged goals of these vaccines? Transhumanism, eugenics, new world order, depopulation of earth? It is all that. It is said that 1,700 vaccinated people die per day in Indonesia. The internationally renowned immunologist, Mr. Mike Yeedon, former chief scientist of Pfizer, says that "Immediately after the first vaccination, about 0.8% of people die within two weeks." What is the International Criminal Court doing in the face of this planetary genocide? Nobel Prize winner Luc Montagnier confirmed that there was no chance of survival for people who received any form of the covid-19 vaccine. He said bluntly: "There is no hope and no cure for those who have been vaccinated. We must be prepared to cremate the bodies ". It is the vaccination that creates the variants. Note that in the United States, the Supreme Court canceled universal vaccination. Bill Gates, the American infectious disease specialist, Fauci and Big Pharma lost a lawsuit in the United States Supreme Court, failing to prove that all of their vaccines in the past 32 years were safe for health citizens! The lawsuit was filed by a group of scientists led by Senator Kennedy.

For the first time in the history of vaccination, the so-called latest generation mRNA vaccines directly interfere with the genetic material of the patient and therefore alter the individual genetic material which is genetic manipulation, which was already prohibited and was previously considered to be a crime. The corona virus vaccine is not a vaccine! Warning! What has always been a vaccine? It was always the pathogen itself, a microbe or a virus that was killed or suppressed, that is to say weakened, and it was introduced into the body in order to produce antibodies. This is not the case for so-called anti-covid vaccines.

APPENDICES

Suzanne Celeste Delaunay Belleville

Response Letter To Be Vaccinated

Dear,

I have received the invitation to receive an mRNA vaccine against SARS-Cov-2 and thank you for it.

Before taking any related decision, I would like you to inform me (1) by replying to me in writing (2) on the following points which seem fundamental to me:

1. Give me the complete list of the ingredients of the vaccines currently in circulation in our country;
2. Certify that the vaccine you plan to inject me does not contain MRCS (cells from aborted fetuses or traces of human DNA), which would go against my religious convictions;
3. Certify to me that there is no risk of introgenic reactions;
4. Inform me of all the contraindications and all the potential side effects, repairable or irreparable, in the short, medium and long term;
5. Certify unequivocally and in good faith, in compliance with article 13 of the Oviedo Convention (3), that this technology does not have the potential to modify human DNA thanks to what called reverse transcriptase, which explicitly allows the transfer of information from mRNA to DNA;
6. Certify that this vaccine does not contain HIV virus inserts;
7. Certify that the vaccine does not contain any Radio Frequency Identification (Rfid) chip or nano-technology in any form;
8. Certify to me that all the medical parameters concerning the required tests and studies have been met;
9. Tell me what are the other possible treatments to fight against SARS-Cov-2 by detailing the advantages and disadvantages of each treatment within the meaning of article 2 of the Nuremberg Code (4).

In addition, please give me a simple yes or no answer to the following questions:

1. If I get vaccinated, can I stop wearing a mask?
2. If I get the vaccine, can I stop social distancing?
3. If I get vaccinated, do I still have to adhere to the curfew?
4. If my parents, grandparents and I are all vaccinated, can we hug each other again?
5. If I get vaccinated, will I be resistant to covid and its many variants and for how long?
6. If I get vaccinated, will I avoid severe forms with hospitalization, as well as death?
7. If I get the vaccine, will I be contagious to others?
8. If I experience a serious adverse reaction, long-term (as yet unknown) effects that even lead to death, will I (or my family) be compensated?

On the other hand, in addition to your answers, I intend to inform myself in a contradictory way by the indications given by the laboratories and the official experts of the Government, but also by independent scientists and the testimonies of people who have already been vaccinated. It means that only when I have collected all this information, I will be able to give you my free and informed consent (5), after having objectively assessed the benefit / risk balance.

If necessary, I will come back to you, possibly having selected the vaccine that would suit me best. I am in perfect health and have no intention of traveling, which allows me to take a step back in order to make a thoughtful and responsible decision, always having in mind the Hippocratic Oath which remains the founding stone of our medicine: "Primum non nocere".

Legal references

(1) "I will properly inform the people who call for my care. Hippocratic Oath, version adapted by the National Council of the Order of Physicians (July 2011)

(2) "Law of 22 August 2002 on the rights of the patient-article 7, paragraph 2:" Communication with the patient takes place in a clear language. The patient can request that the information be confirmed in writing.

SIDE EFFECTS OF COVID-19 VACCINES

According to several testimonies collected around the world, here are some unwanted side effects of vaccines:

1. headache
2. fainting
3. lost memory
4. sight loss
5. chest pain
6. inability to urinate
7. heart attack
8. inability to eat
9. inability to speak
10. inability to walk
11. vomiting
12. The mobile phone remains stuck to the arm, without falling, when it is placed on it. The body of the vaccinee has become like a magnet that sucks and holds the cell phone.

Bioethics

Bioethics is a reflection on the progress of research in the fields of biology, medicine and health. This neologism born in the 1970s thus brings together the ethical or moral questions posed by these technological or scientific advances and the impact they can have on human beings. It ranges from the medicine-patient relationship to the broader questions posed by public health and the humanities, as well as ecological issues such as climate change. It is thus a matter of joint work at the crossroads of several disciplines: science, philosophy, law, medicine, ethics. Bioethics invites us to reflect on the possible drifts that scientific progress can engender and also to reflect on the limits to be set to prevent man from harming his neighbor. It is an arbiter or a bridge between research, medicine and society. For bioethics, scientific and technological efficiency does not imply law, legitimacy, morality.

GAVI

It's the World Vaccine Alliance. It is an organization whose mission is to improve access to vaccines for the world's most vulnerable children. Founded in 2000, its goal is to save lives, fight poverty and protect the world from the threat of epidemics.

GAVI acts in partnership with the public and private sectors to carry out its mission. It collaborates with non-profit organizations, organizations and pressure groups, governments, vaccine manufacturers, researchers etc. so as to improve access to vaccines in all settings.

"The world needs GAVI now more than ever, both to ensure that covid-19 vaccines reach all countries, rich and poor, and to continue its core mission of protecting hundreds of millions of people against preventable diseases, "said Jose Manuel Barroso, quoted in a GAVI press release.

This Alliance brings together low-income countries and donor governments, WHO, UNICEF, the World Bank, vaccine manufacturers from various countries, technical and research institutes, civil society, the Bill and Melinda Gates Foundation and other private philanthropists.

Since the covid-19 pandemic, the Geneva-based organization has been tasked by the World Health Organization with coordinating the UN system for global access to the vaccine against covid-19, called Covax (covid-19 Vaccine Global Access; global access to covd-19 vaccine). The board of directors of GAVI - where UNICEF, WHO, the World Bank and the Bill and Melinda Gates Foundation occupy permanent seats - unanimously approved the choice of the former Prime Minister of Portugal (2002 -2004), who headed the European Commission for ten years (2004-2014) before working for the investment bank Goldman Sachs.

GAVI plays a key role in the fight against the new coronavirus pandemic. This public-private partnership, created in 2000 to expand access to immunization in poor countries, currently oversees the UN system for global access to the vaccine against covid-19.

GSK

Glaxo Smithkline (GSK) is a British multinational, one of the ten giants of the global pharmaceutical industry.

AMT

In 1997, the World Transhumanist Association (AMT) was founded with the objective of transforming transhumanism into an academic discipline ... Transhumanism is more than the abstract belief that we are about to transcend our biological limits by through technology; it is also an attempt to reassess the complete situation of the human being as traditionally perceived. The transhumanists invite people to take a constructive approach and a long-term view to our new condition. Those who want the human condition to be a **constant** are not transhumanists. Calling nature or the human condition into question, making it evolve, progress (change, improvement) is transhumanism. Modern technologies such as genetic engineering, information technology, pharmaceutical medicine as well as the anticipation of future capacities including nano-technology, artificial intelligence, downloading of brain data into a computer or uploding, perpetual bliss by chemical modification (paradise engineering) and the colonization of space are part of the sphere of interest of transhumanists. According to Nick Bostrom.

Transhumanism

Transhumanism is an interdisciplinary approach that leads us to understand and assess the avenues that will allow us to **overcome our biological limits through technological progress**. Transhumanists seek to develop technical possibilities so that people live longer and in good health while increasing their intellectual, physical and emotional capacities (elitism and eugenics).

New technologies raise important fundamental scientific, social and ethical questions. The World Transhumanist Association was founded to encourage discussion, research and increase the visibility of transhumanist thought among the public.

Nick Bostrom

Department of Philosophy, Logic and Scientific Methodology London School of Economics.

Book Summary

This book is part of the critical thinking called **bioethics** (anti-scientism) or critical philosophy with regard to the progress of the science of life and technology harmful to humanity. The science of life, technology and progressive philosophy, eugenics, transhumanists and globalists (new world order) lead men to collective suicide or planetary genocide. It is about the suppression of humanity and civilization in favor of barbarism and chaos beneficial to businessmen, political leaders, madmen, wizards, satanists and all those they have corrupted and instrumentalised. This book is a vibrant appeal to the living. **This is my heartfelt cry against the macabre logic and dynamics of transhumanist covidism.**

AUTHOR'S BIOGRAPHY

François Adja Assemien, alias Dr Kamamo, was born on March 15, 1954, in Côte d'Ivory. He studied humanities (Latin and Greek), human sciences and philosophy. He is graduate in philosophy (PhD) and sociology (Bachelor's degree). He devoted himself to teaching philosophy, writing, academic research and journalism. He speaks and writes three modern languages: French, English and German.

He is author of several works published in English and French (novels, essays, tales, plays) and of several concepts such as Afrocratism, African conscience, philocure, sidarology, abubu music... He is also an artist, musician, composer, singer and guitarist. He lives in the United States of America.

www.ingramcontent.com/pod-product-compliance
Lightning Source LLC
Chambersburg PA
CBHW022042050726
47591CB00003B/910